My Secrets to Regaining Health

Thank you for your purchase.

We hope this book gives you insights for a healthier, happier life.
What a great gift for family, friends and health practitioners!

Pay it forward!
Please write a short book review at Amazon.com so that others can be helped.
We are grateful for recommendations of our book.

Thank you.

DR. IDELLE BRAND

Disclaimer

The author of this book does not dispense medical advice or prescribe the use of any technique as a form of treatment for physical or medical problems. Please consult with a physician directly. The intent of the author is only to offer information of a general nature to help you in your quest for emotional and physical well being. In the event that you use any of the information in this book for yourself, which is your constitutional right, the author and the publisher assume no responsibility for your action.

When we do what we need to do
learn what we need to learn
only then
we will become who we are meant to be.
        --Enlightened Indigo Child

ACKNOWLEDGEMENTS

Many thanks to my amazing patients
who have given me inspiration and hope
when all seemed lost.

CONTENTS

INTRODUCTION

*The world is full of suffering. It is also full of
overcoming it.*
            -Helen Keller

Being healthy has always been a main aspiration for
me. So when I was diagnosed with chronic Lyme
disease with no foreseeable cure, I decided it was
time to take matters into my own hands.

The year was 1994. I already had Lyme for 2 years,
getting progressively weaker and sicker. During those
two years, I had seen many doctors with no definitive
diagnosis. Other than a recommendation of seeing a
psychiatrist for my undiagnosable psychosomatic
"fake" symptoms, there was nothing that could be
done.

Believe me; I had all the tests and scans with all the
experts, including a spinal tap (ouch), MRI and CAT
scans, which all came up negative.

By the time I was properly diagnosed, I was, to put it
mildly, a vegetable. Brain fog was the new normal,
along with cardiac arrhythmias, tremors, extreme
muscle weakness (my legs could not support me),

MY SECRETS TO REGAINING HEALTH

intestinal issues, and a host of other daunting symptoms too numerous to list.

Treatment with proper antibiotics and medications was the next step, with small breakthroughs here and there, but ultimately, the illness prevailed. Eight years later, I had finally rid myself of this complicated disease, but many symptoms still lingered. The road back to health was slow and at times, hopeless.

But here I am today, healthier now than I have ever been. This book holds many of the secrets that I have learned. Use this guide as a base and expand from here.

On this journey, I have learned that the solutions to impossible health challenges do indeed exist. They just don't always come neatly wrapped up and presented to you by the physician. Doctors are important, but ultimately, you hold the answers to your own health matters.

After all, no one knows you as well as you know you. Do not accept a medical diagnosis by "experts" as a defining limitation for your health. Medical miracles happen every day, and you may just be the next one.

Your body is like an entire pharmacy just waiting to send out the right hormones, neurotransmitters and other chemicals to heal you. You must believe in your inner ability to heal yourself.

You were born healthy and when you once again find

that balance in your body to heal, you will be healthy again. Remove the toxins, rebuild the immune system and change your entire paradigm of what modern medicine is. Your health will shift. Mine did. And yours can too.

HEALTHY HOME

Where there is love there is life.
    –Mahatma Gandhi

Contaminants are found everywhere; our food, air, shelter and even medicines. Unless you live in the wilderness, grow your own food and meditate daily, it is difficult to avoid them.

We spend much of our life in our own homes; houses and apartments full of exasperating people and lots of dangerous chemicals. Disconnected from nature, this can be a fairly toxic environment, emotionally and physically.

There have always been frequent warnings about toxins in our environment. Some we have control over; most we don't.   Therefore we must do all we can to protect ourselves as best we can in our own home.

When you add material toxins to an unhappy home life (family arguments, abuse), you can really develop some major health issues. So it is very important that we do as much as possible for our own protection.

Many of the topics that I discuss here are fairly general and can be applied to anyone, regardless of their particular health concerns. Creating improved well-being and mental harmony should be a goal in every household.

▪ De-stress your home

How people treat you is their karma; how you react is yours.
　　　　　-Dr. Wayne Dyer

There is a need for a healthy emotional home environment for a person to be well. This means no screaming, yelling, cursing, hitting or belittling allowed. Not at your spouse, child, pet or neighbor. This may be easier said than done, as we have very little control over other's actions.

If this distressing kind of behavior is commonplace in your home, then imbalance, frustration, anger, depression, emotional and mental illness may manifest. Physical illness will soon follow.

Living in this type of environment, it may be extremely difficult to regain your health. This low frequency energy of anger or depression will build on itself continuing to make you unbalanced on the physical, mental and emotional planes.

These are the simplest do-it-yourself options that I recommend to release emotional stress.

1. **Keep a journal.** Journal writing means that you write down your thoughts and experiences on a regular basis. This will help you keep track of your own emotional growth as a person. It will also help you to release some pent up emotions and to clarify your personal health or life goals.

2. **Write a letter.** This is your opportunity to get everything off your chest. Write exactly how you are feeling in a letter to the person that upset you. Include everything; details, events and even profanity if needed. It all has to come out. This is helpful to get these emotions out of your head and onto the paper. Pinpoint who you are angry at. Explain why you're angry, how you feel about this person and any other things you may wish to say to their face but can't.

   Once you are done writing all you need to write, you need to end the letter with the words "I forgive you."

   Forgiveness is a difficult emotion to express when someone has hurt you. But it is needed so that you can move on. If you do not forgive that person, they will always have power over you and be able to manipulate you emotionally.

Finally, you must destroy the letter. Yes, you read that correctly – destroy the letter. It will not do you or the other person any good if they actually read it. If anything, it will probably incite them again and escalate the bad emotions to an even more dangerous level. The best way to destroy the letter is to burn it, rip it into a million pieces, bury it or throw it in the garbage.

If you find that any emotion continues to come up again, then you can write them another letter elaborating on the further details of your angst. Again, you must destroy the letter.

3. **Send love.** The frequency of love is very powerful. Even though you might be feeling hate for this person, feeling more hate does not improve the circumstance. As many of us already know, hate is really not the emotion in question here. It is really the absence of love.

Healthy Home

*If we really want to love, we must
learn how to forgive.*
–Mother Teresa

You need to elevate the situation to a
higher frequency by putting them in
imaginary white light and then send them
love. This may be an emotionally tough
thing to do if you haven't done #2 first.

To send them love can be done simply by
surrounding them with imaginary hearts
or angels, or even having a cute puppy
playing with them. You can even envision
them as a baby being cuddled by their
mommy.

Basically imagine anything that resonates
for you. It is the intention that makes this
technique work, not the actual imagery.
You must feel it in your heart as real as
you can possibly make it. If you find it
tough to send them this love energy, it will
be helpful if you ground yourself (connect
to nature) and send love to your own self
first. Then when you are feeling more at
ease, try sending love to them. That should
do it.

Do this exercise for at least 10 minutes or longer. You will notice the shift. Not only in you, but in the other person as well.

4. **Feel gratitude.** Just like love, gratitude is a high frequency. Having gratitude for the positive memories, lessons learned, and experiences you have, is one step closer to forgiveness.

Say or think the sentence: *I am grateful for_____.*

Just fill in the blank. Do this exercise as often as you can for as long as you can; for at least ten minutes or longer. It almost becomes a form of meditation and can create an inner peace like no medication could ever possibly achieve.

I often use this as a walking meditation:

"What beautiful trees. Thank you trees for being here and cleaning our air and making the street lovelier. .....What a beautiful building. So tall and majestic. Wow. And look at that pretty architecture. ..... The clouds. They're so puffy and white. Thank you for providing rain for the

plants to grow and giving us water to drink..... And look at that beautiful big pile of garbage on the street. Somebody just cleaned out their home to make room for new stuff......And those dirty pots and dishes left in the sink. So grateful to have such healthy food to eat on these lovely dishes."

You get the point. Find the joy of everything. It's there if you change your paradigm viewpoint.

While the old adage says to count sheep if you can't sleep, I say to count blessings. Not only will you fall asleep quicker, you will be in a very restful high frequency state of tranquility. Your dreams will be better and you will wake up more refreshed than ever. The added bonus is that you will see your life attracting more positive experiences. It's a paradigm shift of focusing on what you have and not on what you want or don't have. You are using the _Universal Law of Attraction_ to attract more of whatever you think about.

If you worry incessantly on how a particular person is mean, guess what? They will be.

But if you feel gratitude for all the nice things they have done (given you shelter, helped you with paying bills, etc.) then you will find that they may continue to do more of it.

5. **Be grounded.** When you are grounded, you are able to think clearer and are able to forgive.

    Hold on to a house plant, rock or crystal. Walk barefoot on the grass or beach. Hug a tree. When you connect to the Earth and resonate with her energy, you will find yourself in a natural flow of life and less likely to get upset. You will also be able to think clearer.

    There is a lot to be said about grounding, and by far this may be the single most important thing to do to reclaim your mind, health and power.

    It is important to note that there is an excess number of free electrons on the earth's surface. You, on the other hand, are full of free radicals. When you physically connect to the planet, the earth's free electrons will flow to you, attach to the free radicals and neutralize them. This makes nature the greatest antioxidant in the world. And it costs nothing.

6. **Walk.** Walking is a great exercise. Besides giving you a change of scenery, it will also help you let off some steam through the production of endorphins (the happy hormone). The more you walk, the better you will feel mentally and emotionally. When you take a walk, the new environment will give you a new perspective on any situation. Walk to a place that will give you peace; there's the park, pet store or library.

Parks are a great place that you can connect with nature and ground yourself. As you gaze at the trees, grass, flowers and wildlife, your mood can't help but shift. If you rub your bare feet and hands into the grass, you will find that your tension is releasing. Sit there for at least twenty minutes.

If you have a pet, take it for a walk, read to it, and play with it. Animals are so naturally grounded since they always walk barefoot on the earth. So if you can hold a pet, you will find your energy shifting.

Even window shopping can be transformative. Just don't buy anything as this may create regret or upset later.

7. **Use your imagination or read a book.** If written well, books can quickly help lift you out of your distressed mood. Libraries are filled with resources. The wonderful part about books is that they take you on a journey. They allow you to live other people's lives and teach you how to navigate in our world.

   Get involved in creative projects. Music, art, dance and sports are a wonderful release and distraction from day to day annoyances. Just do not use it as an escape from your home situation. Creative projects are there to keep you in balance.

   By the way, watching television is NOT using your imagination.

8. **Breathe.** Deep breathing is so often overlooked. The deeper you breathe the more oxygen will go throughout your body. This will give you a chance to relax, as it releases tension and elevates your mood.

Your mind will clear and allow you to rethink what should be the next step. Try to inhale into the base of your abdomen. This way you know that you will be using maximum lung capacity and will receive maximum oxygen supply throughout your body. And when your cells get more oxygen, you will become calmer. Not to mention you will even improve your physical and mental health.

9. **Meditate.** Find the quiet within. Focus on the positive. See and feel yourself already healed. Resonate that energy through you. The cells will pick up on this new vibration. They will reproduce at a healthier energy level. You will feel stronger and your mind will be clearer.

   Every cell of your body is totally replaced within 12 months. Start now and give them the proper vibrational frequency to be healthier. Daily meditation is key.

Bottom line: It is always paramount that you get yourself out of the space where the offensive person is. It is also best not to respond to the person if what they are saying is negative. If you have an irresistible urge to respond, then simply say: "Thank you for sharing." Smile and walk away.

This sentence, "Thank you for sharing," is used to defuse the situation. You are acknowledging the person but are basically responding with something neutral to what they say. It's active listening at its best. Acknowledge them, but don't get involved. Your health depends on it.

When you are angry, upset, sad, or depressed, your body will not heal. Apply the techniques in the above list. You will become calmer and the situation will be transmuted from a harmful state to a higher frequency of healing.

Problem people do not have to be problems. They present challenges for us, so it is imperative to tap into our own wisdom and do whatever is necessary to protect ourselves and shift the situation.

Only *you* have complete control of *your* emotions. Do not let others push your buttons.

Always seek less turbulent skies.
Hurt.
Fly above it.
Betrayal.
Fly above it.
Anger.
Fly above it.

You are the one who is flying the plane.
    -Marianne Williamson

▪ **Detoxify your home**

Home is where the heart is.
        -Gaius Plinius Secundas

It is important to keep in mind that we are all
assaulted by hundreds, if not thousands of toxic
materials from our environment every day. Most are
insidious, hidden in food, medicines, air, and
invisible sound waves. We can't hide ourselves in a
plastic bubble all day and night, but we can take
control and start removing the ones that are
obvious.

Sick building syndrome is not just for people who
work in poorly ventilated office buildings.
According to the World Health Organization, up to
30% of new and remodeled buildings worldwide
may be linked to this syndrome. But it is also
present in older buildings as well.

It usually comes down to flaws in heating,
ventilation or air conditioning. Other contributing
factors include the outgassing of volatile organic
compounds (VOC) like formaldehyde and plastics
from new construction materials (new carpeting is
really bad), mold or inordinate amounts of dust, dirt

and animal hairs.

Since moving from your home may be impossible, here is a checklist of what you can do to lessen the toxicity in your home:

- Keep your house as clean as possible. Dust and vacuum daily. Change the bed linens at least twice a week. Remove all carpeting. Not only does carpeting outgas, it also collects tons of dirt in the microfibers that you are breathing in constantly. Adverse health effects suffered by carpet installers are a clear-cut way to see the hazards of this product. Most documented are neurological problems and higher rates of cancer. If you must have carpet, make sure that it is as natural as possible.

- Use natural cleaners. Replace chemical cleaners with essential oils, baking soda and vinegar. Tea tree oil is especially effective at removing mold and mildew. Baking soda acts as an abrasive to remove stains and residue from glass, ceramic and stainless steel. You can add a few drops of water to make a paste to clean the stove, sink, tub or toilet. White vinegar is excellent as a window and mirror cleaner. Add your favorite essential oil if you want a pleasant smell.

Recipe for an easy non-toxic all purpose

cleaner: 1 cup white vinegar, 5 drops tea tree oil, 5 drops lavender oil, ½ cup water. Mix in a labeled spray bottle. That's it. It is great to use on counters, and stove tops. It is not meant for porous surfaces such as wood. It costs pennies to make and even the most sensitive person will have virtually no perceptible reaction. You can use less water to make it stronger.

As a side note to this, you should avoid all artificially fragranced products: air fresheners, household cleaners, detergents. Unscented may very well be a highly processed product. It takes a lot of chemicals to mask a smell, so fragrance-free may be toxic chemical-full. Fluffer sheets used in the dryer can be more toxic than your detergent. Use the silicone dryer balls instead. Plus it is much more cost effective, as they have an infinite reusable lifespan. As always, read ingredient lists carefully to make sure your product is as natural as possible.

- Remove plastic from your eating arsenal. If you have any plastic dishes or cups, throw them out. Bis phenyl A (BPA) is a known xenoestrogen and will affect the hormone balance of your body. Besides its known carcinogenic effect, it will also create imbalance within your endocrine system and ultimately affect mental and physical vigor. Leaking of bis phenyl A into your water from plastic bottles has already been documented. And the longer the water has been in the bottle, the more BPA you will be ingesting.

Xenoestrogen is one of the most troubling types of endocrine disruptors. It will mimic estrogen and attach to the body's estrogen-receptor sites; in both sexes (notice men are developing breast overgrowth). These xenoestrogens interfere with hormonal signaling and are believed to cause an increased risk of hormonal imbalances contributing to breast, prostate, and reproductive cancers; reduced fertility; early puberty in children; menstrual irregularities; endometriosis; numerous cysts and other disorders.

Here is an informative BPA story from my own experience.

An interesting occurrence just happened with our dog Celeste. She has pretty much always eaten from stainless steel bowls. But about 6 months ago, we started serving her home cooked food from the plastic container that it was stored in, in the refrigerator. She developed a little growth on her lip. The veterinarian said that Celeste probably bit herself and a little fibroma formed. Then about 3 weeks ago, part of her nose started changing color from black to pinkish white. This time we went online to see if we could find the answers ourselves. Not wanting to buy into the gloom and doom of my dog being old (she's 3) or has a weird skin condition or blame it on the weather (hard to believe but seasonal change will cause this shift), we looked further. There was something we found about chemicals in plastic dishes possibly creating the color change. We figured this would be a simple thing to correct. We immediately changed all her serving bowls back to stainless or ceramic. Guess what? In three days, not only was her nose changing back to normal color but that growth on her lip was also disappearing. One week later, there was no trace of any dis-ease on her nose or lip. My beautiful healthy puppy had her baby face back.

Thank you Celeste for that personal real life

lesson on the dangers of plastics in our environment. The thing to realize is that Celeste is a 12 pound dog. The effects on her were visually seen. If you are a 100 or 150 pound person, the effects will not be so obvious. However, you should know that theses toxins are accumulating in your body, and affecting every part of you- skin, hair, brain, and especially your hormone systems that control everything. Plastics have chemicals that will act like hormones and this will throw your whole body out of whack.

Celeste has a very clean healthy diet, so her body immediately threw the toxins to the skin surface in an attempt to remove them. I doubt that us humans will be that lucky. It will take a bit more effort than that.

- Do not use the microwave. Microwave ovens are radiation ovens. When you say it like that, the reality of this machine is clear. The microwave radiation distorts the molecular structure of the foods; it destroys much of the nutrients and causes many problems with the immune system. If you value your health, take the extra couple of minutes to heat the food up the right way.

- Limit cell phone use. Cell phones expose us to a form of electromagnetic radiation frequency (EMF). Scientists have suspected that this radiation might increase the risk of brain cell damage leading to tumors, and in 1995 they found this to be the case in rats. An analysis of the most rigorous studies found convincing evidence linking the use of handheld phones to brain tumors, especially in users of a decade or longer. Regardless of brain tumors, we personally know of people who feel physically ill when using the cell phone. It affects brainwaves. That's enough information for me. Use it sparingly and stick to the land line (NOT cordless) as much as possible. Buy an EMF protector and install it on your cell phone.

- Limit computer use. Besides the obvious eye and wrist strain, there is a generating of EMFs. Nobody would sit at a desk under high voltage power lines. Yet we will happily sit a foot away from a computer screen, with a computer and printer on the desk next to us, and perhaps even a power supply near our feet. The old box-shaped cathode-ray tube (CRT) computer monitors generally have quite high levels of radiation. Best to invest in a flat screen monitor. And of course EMF protectors are essential.

- Limit television watching or better yet, remove it completely from the home.

Research shows that your brain literally shifts into a passive state when you're watching television. Experiencing "brain fog" is not uncommon. Your alpha brain waves increase after television exposure.

Alpha waves are commonly associated with a relaxed meditative state as well as brain states associated with suggestibility. You can achieve a good alpha state through meditation – and that can be an active process producing insight and calm. Too much time spent in the low alpha wave state caused by TV can cause unfocussed daydreaming and inability to concentrate. Researchers have said that watching television is similar to staring at a blank wall or sitting in a dark room for several hours.

Aside from this induced state of brain wave altering, most shows are advertisement driven with subliminal messages. And because of this suggestibility state that you are already in, you are more likely to watch shows that are violent or inappropriate for a healthy positive state of mind.

- Remove electronics from the bedroom, especially TV, computers, radio alarm clocks. Again they release a continual dose of EMFs. And if they must be present, then they should be as far away from your head as possible when sleeping and as close to the floor as possible.

- Remove your shoes before coming into your home. Tracking in dirt and germs from outside into the home should be avoided.

- Discard all aluminum or Teflon based cookware. Aluminum will leach into your food. It is a known neurotoxin, causing brain degeneration. Teflon or stick free cookware will eventually chip and enter your food. Better to use high quality stainless steel, cast iron or titanium.

- Do not use aluminum or plastic wrap on foods. And definitely do not microwave anything in or covered with plastic. I usually wrap foods in wax paper first and then outside wrap this with foil or plastic wrap.

- Invest in an air purifier and negative ionizer to eliminate air borne toxins – mold spores, dust, cigarette smoke, pet hair, hydrocarbon toxins and remnants of chemtrails from outside that we may be carrying into our homes.

- Remove fluoride from your intake. This includes toothpastes, mouthwashes, fluoride rinses and municipal drinking water.

The government first began encouraging

municipal water systems to add fluoride in the early 1950s. Since then, fluoride has been put in toothpaste and mouthwash. It is also in a lot of municipal tap waters, bottled waters, and all drinks and foods made from them, including soda, reconstituted juices and baked goods. Additionally, some children may even be prescribed fluoride supplements.

Since 1962, the fluoridated water standard has been in a range of 0.7 parts per million for warmer climates where people drink more water, to 1.2 parts per million in cooler regions. To add insult to injury, 1% – 5% of the population is intolerant to fluoride. These people do not experience an allergic reaction (although that is what the government calls it) but a poisoning reaction. Sodium fluoride has been used for decades as a rat poison and insecticide.

As a result there has been a fluoride overdosing. The most obvious marker for this is in the increase in discoloration found in newly erupted teeth. The less obvious marker is the acknowledged deterioration of brain function. It has already been documented that sodium fluoride is a neurotoxin. Specifically, it will directly affect the pineal gland which in turn will reduce melatonin production. Decrease in melatonin will definitely give you challenges with falling and staying asleep.

Fluoride has also been shown to affect the endocrine system, cause bone fluorosis, cancer and ovarian problems. Thyroid dysfunction is the other big issue since fluoride will disrupt the iodine receptors. It is no surprise that hypothyroidism is widespread.

Just look at a tube of toothpaste and read the warning.

WARNING: Keep out of the reach of children under 6 years of age. If you accidentally swallow more than used for brushing, get medical help or contact a Poison Control Center right away.

I think this label pretty much puts a lid on the topic. No more to say other than, "Why would anyone put this stuff in their mouth?" Goodness knows that if it's in your mouth, you are going to swallow some of it. It's just not possible not to.

As a side thought, it might be wise to

purposely request *no fluoride treatments* for you and your children at dental visits. Just because it comes highly recommended and insurance companies will pay for it, that doesn't mean it's good for you. Even if you receive it for free from your dental insurance carrier, that doesn't make this poison any less toxic. As a practicing dentist for many decades, I have heard several stories of young children dying from an acute fluoride overdose in the dental office. Do not let you or your child become a statistic.

Now, what do you do if it's in the municipal tap water, and all the drinks and foods made from it? It's pretty scary when you start thinking about how much fluoride you are really consuming.

It is important to note that fluoride safety has never been approved by the FDA. *Fluoride ingestion does not reduce tooth decay.* Its predominant anti-caries effect is topical, not systemic. And certainly there are safer ways to prevent cavities than the use of fluoride. (How about cutting down the frequency of sugary sticky foods? Or rinsing your mouth with plain water after you eat them?).

The bottom line is that the water supply should not be used as a drug delivery system to individuals without regard to age, weight, health, need, and informed consent.

Fluoride is the only water additive intended to treat people and not the water.

It may not be long before the cities routinely start adding other chemicals to treat people. There has already been talk of adding trace amounts of Lithium to our water to suppress bipolar, manic depressant disorder and suicide.

- Invest in a water purifier. City water is loaded with chemicals to make it potable. I have a double carbon and alumina filter installed under my sink. You may need a plumber to install it, but it is definitely worth the expense. Not only does the water taste cleaner, but you are actually getting quality water that will help your body detoxify properly, instead of poisoning it even more.

Bottled spring water is not the answer, as this will only give you toxins from the plastic containers. It is much easier to actively work at omitting these toxins from our life instead of waiting to see if we get sick from them. By the time we notice the effect upon us, there will be so many adverse and diverse symptoms that it may be almost impossible to regain our health. It is not just an issue of removing toxins from our bodies but also an issue of rebuilding our bodies from that damaged point. It takes years to get sick, and it will probably take just as long to regain health.

Other options beside the carbon and alumina filters would include installing a reverse osmosis filter or a water distiller to remove everything that's not water. You might have to add some mineral salts back to the water so that you do not become mineral deficient. Most pitcher water filters are carbon filters. They are better than nothing but they will not remove fluoride.

As a side note, boiling water does not remove toxins. It will just kill living organisms (bacteria, parasites, mold, etc.) that may be present. Chemical toxins will still be present. Also, for those energetically aware, the life force of the water will be lowered considerably. So if you are going to make any hot beverage, best to heat the water to right below the boiling temperature.

- Consider having your home tested for mold, radon and lead.

- Replace vinyl (PVC) blinds. They are quite popular as inexpensive window coverings but also quite toxic. They release massive byproducts of hydrochloric acid, vinyl chloride, mercury, cadmium, lead and an extremely dangerous carcinogen, dioxin.

- Add plants to your home. Not only will they help keep you grounded energetically, they will also clean the air you breathe. Some easily found varieties such as spider plant, snake plant, English ivy and Boston fern are known to filter harmful chemicals. Make sure that the plants you bring into your home are not poisonous to your pets.

- Clean out all air ducts and vents regularly. Investigate the use of furnace filters. Be sure that a carbon monoxide detector is up in your home so that you are not breathing this insidious noxious odorless gas.

- Open windows regularly. Indoor air pollution is always more dangerous than outdoor air pollution, even in busy industrialized cities.

MY SECRETS TO REGAINING HEALTH

By integrating just one of these techniques into your life and maintaining it, your life will change for the better, dramatically. The ability to think clearer and sleep better should be obvious within a few weeks, if not sooner. Prevention is worth more than a pound of cure. Get started today.

HEALTHY BODY

A happy, healthy, vibrant, passionate, fulfilling life is available to you right now - all you need to do is to decide that you want it! - Gary Null, PhD

I remember seeing the movie *Lorenzo's Oil* many years ago that left a deep impression on my soul. It is based on the true story of two parents in a relentless search for a cure for their son Lorenzo's incurable genetic illness. Although conventional medicine had said no cure was possible since it would take years of research and thousands of dollars before they would even be close to finding one, the parents persevered. Through self education, they found the cure. Not giving up is critical to succeeding in regaining your health.

There are many factors contributing to your chronic dis-ease. And most of them, as we have mentioned before, you are probably not even aware of. Not all of these factors are physical toxins.

• **Detoxify your emotions**

Do one thing every day that scares you.
        -Eleanor Roosevelt

Sometimes, it may take a lot of suffering to get us out of our comfort zone. Even with an incurable chronic illness, we can become lazy, almost docile, and just take what conventional medicine dictates. If you are really determined to heal, then now may be the time to make drastic changes in your mindset and do whatever is needed, even if your family and doctors frown upon it. This is your life, and ultimately you are the one responsible for it.

* * *

As we discussed in a previous section, it is difficult to regain health if we are carrying the memory of emotional traumas. It is a good bet that not all of these traumas are from your present situation.

You have had an entire lifetime to experience disturbing emotional events, many of which you have long since forgotten about or repressed. This could very well be the unyielding foundation for your chronic health issues that won't resolve.

A good example of this would be if you had a chronic stiff shoulder because some teacher grabbed you there when you were 6 years old and said a negative comment about how bad you were at the time. Since you can't go back and have closure with this particular person, there are other ways to resolve and release this trauma.

1. As is standard, see a competent therapist for guidance and support. To bring this one step further, consider seeing practitioners of EFT (Emotional Freedom Technique) and NLP (NeuroLinguistic Programming). By tapping on critical meridian points or reframing traumatic events, an entire experience can be released. Many times this is almost instant, taking no more than a few moments. Once this emotional weight is lifted, you will feel amazingly lighter, happier and healthier. So it is definitely worth investigating and finding an experienced practitioner to work with.

2. Consider seeing an Energy Healer. There are many modalities of Energy Medicine, so if one type doesn't work, another might. Craniosacral Therapy, Homeopathy, Reiki, Therapeutic Touch, are several examples of this. Personally, I was able to release the pain of fibromyalgia (of 12 years duration) by taking a weekend course in Sound Therapy.

I have also had great success by working with a intuitive metaphysical healer. She was able to realign my energy field by releasing stagnant energy and channeling in a higher energy for healing.

You should bear in mind that one visit will probably not do it. There are always many layers to releasing emotional traumas. You can also help this process by continuously listening to grounding or high vibrational music in your environment. I have CDs of whale sounds and chakra balancing melodies that keep my office at a high vibration for healing. Many people feel this immediately when they come for their appointments. You should play these in your home, especially while sleeping. It is like getting an eight hour energy treatment. Wow!

The most important thing is to keep an open mind about these alternative types of healing. They are not airy-fairy. All can be explained through quantum physics and real science. Just make sure that your practitioner is competent and comes with some recommendations.

▪ **Detoxify your body**

*To keep the body in good health is a duty, otherwise
we shall not be able to keep our mind strong and
clear.*
>   -Budha

• **Have yourself tested for heavy metals.**

Heavy metal toxicity in today's society is rampant.
As a practicing dentist for over 30 years, and as a
holistic educator, I can honestly say that heavy
metals are probably the number one contributor to
chronic neurological health diseases on the physical
and mental planes. This includes but is not limited
to Autism, Alzheimer's, Parkinson's and Multiple
Sclerosis.

Mercury poisoning has been implicated in a host of
chronic symptoms of dis-ease, so it might be a good
eye opener to have a look at this website:
 http://www.mercurypoisoned.com/symptoms.html
to see if any of the mercury toxicity symptoms
resonate with you.

You may be wondering how you could possibly
have gotten into this situation. It is very easy when
you understand that mercury is present in many
products that we are exposed to routinely.

You remember all those tuna fish sandwiches you
ate as a kid?–toxic mercury (environmental). Or
how about the 22 or so vaccines that you were

exposed to in the first 6 years of your life? - toxic mercury (preservative). Or the shiny silver fillings in your mouth? - toxic mercury.

And if you yourself don't have those silver mercury fillings, how about your mother who carried you for 9 months in utero. Mercury does pass through the placental barrier. That would certainly be enough to get your system exposed to a high loading dose of mercury. And as you grew up, and made your regular checkups for immunizations, your exposure only increased, augmenting the toxic load. The cumulative amount of mercury being given to children in the average number of vaccines by age 6, would be an amount equivalent to 187 times the EPA daily exposure limit!!!!

So now that you know this, you need to take action. If you have been diagnosed with a physical or mental disorder, or if you just don't feel right most of the time, I highly recommend that you be tested for heavy metal toxicity. It is a simple non-invasive urine test that is easily done at any competent physician's office.

Of course, it must be recognized that heavy metal toxicity is not the only cause of all chronic health disorders. However, it can be said that mercury toxicity may be an original trigger and can set off a plethora of symptoms and syndromes. Therefore, if neurological or autoimmune symptoms are present, it is logical to check for the presence of mercury and all heavy metals.

Bear in mind that the toxic load of heavy metals is cumulative. Even if you were healthy 10 years ago, with a similar exposure amount as today, the heavy metal load would have been accumulating throughout the years, slowly doing damage to the cells in your body and overtaxing your immune system. In addition, your immune system has simultaneously been becoming less vital just from normal chronological aging.

Then, when your physical body becomes overburdened, your mental and emotional fields will follow. Diverse symptoms of illness are soon your new normal.

Now would be the ideal time to rule out heavy metal toxicity as the culprit for your chronic health issues. Do the right thing. Get the simple 24 hour urine Heavy Metal Toxicity test and learn if this is the cause of your health challenges.

As an afterthought, there are many physicians who don't have a clue about this particular 24 hour urine Heavy Metal Toxicity test. If your doctor is not familiar with it or not willing to do this kind of heavy metal test, it may be time to find a new physician. Information is all over the internet. You would have to be a closed minded physician to belittle a heavy metal toxicity test and dismiss it as inconsequential. A simple blood test or hair analysis may be helpful but will not be conclusive enough to accurately evaluate heavy metals in your system.

If you have been labeled with a chronic or incurable illness that needs to be medicated for life to be "normal", just remember this:

THERE IS NO ILLNESS CAUSED BY A DEFICIENCY OF ANY DRUG.

Yes, that needs repeating.

THERE IS NO ILLNESS CAUSED BY A DEFICIENCY OF ANY DRUG.

When you realize this and truly believe it, you can begin to heal. You are perfection already. You are only out of balance. If you shift to this new paradigm of thinking, the healing will begin.

- **Have yourself tested for hormone imbalance.**

It is not unusual for an imbalance in hormone levels to affect how we think and behave. Heavy metals, fluoride and xenoestrogens (from pesticides, preservatives and plastics) will affect every endocrine gland in your body. The endocrine glands are the ductless glands that are responsible for secreting hormones directly into the bloodstream. The most obvious endocrine glands affected are the pituitary, pineal and thyroid. But others such as the pancreas (diabetes is on the rise), the adrenals (exhaustion), the ovaries and testes (fertility problems), will also be affected.

The pituitary is the master gland of the body. If it is imbalanced, all the other glands will follow. Your genetics and environment will determine which other organs get the brunt of the imbalance. Directly, it will affect your growth hormones.

The pineal gland sits right behind the Third Eye area (between your two eyes and slightly up on the forehead) in your brain. For centuries the pineal was thought to be vestigial with no function at all. We now know that it has a great impact on the sleep-wake cycle due to its production of melatonin. If you have any intuitive sixth sense capabilities, it is usually through the health of your pineal gland. Fluoride will shut it down very quickly.

The thyroid gland controls how quickly the body uses energy, makes proteins, and the sensitivity of the body to other hormones. It has already been documented that heavy metals, especially mercury will cause hypothyroidism. An underactive thyroid will affect all metabolism functions. Make sure that any thyroid test is comprehensive as most routine blood tests only check the TSH level. T4 must also be evaluated to get an accurate assessment.

- **Get your MTHFR gene tested**

The MTHFR gene provides instructions for making an enzyme called methylenetetrahydrofolate reductase. This enzyme is essential for the homeostasis and normal metabolism of intracellular folate (folic acid or Vitamin B-9).

MTHFR gene mutation has been related to many diseases including cancer, leukemia, fibromyalgia, depression, schizophrenia, migraine with aura, glaucoma, neural tube defects, miscarriages, addictions and cardiovascular disease.

There are over 40 types of mutation possible with this gene, so it is important to rule out this factor in any chronic health condition that doesn't resolve. A support site for further information can be found here: http://mthfr.net/.

- **Eat healthy foods.**

Everyone knows the simple adage: *You are what you eat.*

And for those of us who are very ill, these words resonate on an entirely different level. You cannot eat junk food and expect to feel different than "junky". Some of us can live on fast food and be okay, while others will have intense physical and even psychological reactions to the food we eat.

We know that the energy quality of the food affects our health. Obviously, a meal made with love tastes a lot better than food made with anger. Remember when you went to family Thanksgiving dinners and everybody brought something to the meal. It often tasted better and emotionally felt better than even the most delicious luxurious food from take-out. There is a lot to be said for "Grandma's cooking", even if it was the most simple boring dish around. It was always made with love and you could taste it!

Healthy food is an important key for vigor. If you are dealing with chronic illness, you cannot continue to eat what you have always eaten and expect to regain your hardiness. Even if you think you are eating healthy, trust me, there is still a more healthy diet out there. You just haven't discovered it yet. Adapting a more vegetarian diet, preferably raw, with the addition of superfoods like Goji berry, Reishi mushrooms, chlorophyll rich green juices and deep colorful fruits and vegetables, may make a world of difference. Just keep adding more and more healthy foods to your meals. Eventually the poor Standard American Diet (SAD) foods will be crowded out and gone from your daily intake. Eat foods that are as close to nature as possible. If it comes in a package with a list of ingredients you can't pronounce, or has a shelf life longer than your own life, don't eat it!

By the way, white sugar and flour should be totally gone from your menu. Both, even in small quantities, will continue to deplete your immune system.

Natural sugars are fine; like the ones found in fruit, lucuma, molasses, cane juice, coconut palm sugar, xylitol, grade B maple syrup, and raw honey. Agave may be processed so be careful.

And of course, show gratitude for your food. Give thanks for the plant that grew your veggies, for the animal that created that burger. Say a short blessing or thankful words before you chow down.

More importantly, try to eat organic and local farmers' foods as much as possible. An apple fresh off the tree yesterday is going to have more nutrition and taste better than the apple from 3000 miles and a week's truck ride away.

- **Avoid processed foods**

I would like to reiterate that if it comes in a package with a list of ingredients that you can't pronounce, don't eat it. Nobody wants to eat poisons, even if they taste good. If you can't find tasty real foods in the supermarket, now would be a good time to check out your local health food store to see what a better choice would be. That being said, there are plenty of unwholesome foods even in the health food store, so buyer beware!

Look for raw or whole food clubs in your area. Just *Google* it and see what you find. Find a like minded friend and create your own club. You can be the person who creates *the healthy food cooking club* in your neighborhood. If you don't know what to cook, learn! Have a look at the many *YouTube* videos that show you exactly how to make real food, and try it. There is no excuse for being ignorant to the healthy food revolution, as there are more and more health minded cooking schools now open in many big cities.

Many processed foods have hidden sugars in them. Some can be obvious but many are not. Replace chemicalized food with real food. Simple condiments like table salt have sugar added to make it taste better. If you read the ingredient list on Ketchup, don't be surprised to find that tomatoes are not the first ingredient. We all need to be conscious of what we are putting in our bodies. Yummy tasting additives are not nourishing food. They are there as inexpensive fillers and prolongers of product shelf life. They will not nourish your body, mind or spirit. Quite contrary, they will deplete your health and create imbalance and disease. They will keep you hungry as your body will yearn for real nourishment. Obesity will endure, as you persevere in overeating in an attempt to feed your never-ending hunger.

Our good health depends on us making healthy food choices.

- **Avoid artificial sugars, fats, colors and flavors**.

Buying sugar-free or fat-free foods is not a solution when chemicals are added to replace the missing flavors and textures. If anything, it has already been proven that these artificially flavored foods actually make us hungrier. And the reason is simple: Your body will continue to crave real nutrition from real food. If you are only fed artificial food with artificial "enriched" vitamins added, you will continue to be hungry until fed the nutrients that your body needs and wants.

Besides these artificial ingredients providing no natural nourishment, they are toxic chemicals that are poisoning you, slowly over time.

* * *

Sodium saccharine (Sweet-N-Low) was the first artificial sweetener developed. It was accidentally created in 1879 by a researcher at Johns Hopkins University in Baltimore, when he noticed that a derivative of coal tar he accidentally spilled on his hand tasted sweet. Now more than 125 years later, saccharin is joined by a growing list of artificial sweeteners with varying chemical structures and uses. This includes acesulfame potassium, aspartame (NutraSweet or Equal), sucralose (Splenda), and D-Tagatose (Sugaree). And there's a whole host of new ones on the horizon.

Trans fatty acids (margarine or shortening) or fat substitutes (Simplesse, Oatrim, Olestra), and products fortified by plant based ester compounds are found in most processed foods. Next time you reach for coffee creamer, margarine, crackers, bread, or even your favorite brand of potato chips, flip over the bag and take a look at the ingredients-- if you see hydrogenated or partially hydrogenated oil of any type, you're eating a trans fatty acid. The consequences include increased occurrence of heart disease, sexual dysfunction, weakened immune system, cancer, atherosclerosis, diabetes, intestinal problems, and obesity.

It seems that so much food on our supermarket shelves is marketed specifically to attract our attention. Bright colorful packaging with the words *natural, whole grain* and even *organic*, is no guarantee that the food inside is healthy. The manufacturers and advertisers know this. Always look at the list of ingredients in the small print. You may be surprised at what you actually find in your *heart healthy* food.

* * *

Studies have shown that artificial food colors and artificial flavors are associated with the following conditions: allergies, asthma, behavioral issues, hyperactivity, and ADHD, decreased cognitive function, lowered IQ, cancer and brain tumors.

Food dyes are found in all common foods. Here's a basic list of the ones used most often and their known effects:

- ***Yellow #5***: hyperactivity, eczema/hives, aggressive/violent behavior, asthma, irritability, sleep disturbances/insomnia, increased susceptibility to infection
- ***Yellow #6***: hyperactivity, eczema/hives, asthma, tumors
- ***Red #40:*** cancer, reproductive problems, hyperactivity, allergy type reactions
- ***Red #3:*** tumors, neurochemical and behavioral effects

Artificial flavors are also linked to allergic and behavioral reactions, yet these ingredients are not required to be listed in detail as they're *generally recognized as safe* (GRAS) by the FDA.

* * *

MSG (monosodium glutamate) is a popular flavor enhancer. Found to cause brain damage in laboratory mice, it has been banned from use in baby foods, but is still used in many other foods, processed or from restaurants. It causes common allergic and behavioral reactions including headaches, dizziness, chest pains, depression, and mood swings, and is also a possible neurotoxin.

What many people don't know is that more than 40 different ingredients contain the chemical in monosodium glutamate (processed free glutamic acid) that causes these reactions. The most common ingredients that form this toxic free glutamic acid include: corn starch, corn syrup, modified food starch, dextrose, rice syrup, malt extract, soy sauce, yeast extract, *anything* hydrolyzed, *anything* hydrolyzed protein, *anything* flavors or *anything* flavoring, seasonings, carrageenan, bouillon, broth, stock, maltodextrin, citric acid.

That has got to include the majority of packaged foods at the supermarket. What often fooled me was the term *natural flavorings*, thinking it was a healthy ingredient. Then I found out that this is a euphemism for MSG or aspartame.

READ INGREDIENTS BEFORE BUYING!!!

- **Remove heavy metals and plastics (xenoestrogens) from your diet.**

Whether you have been diagnosed with heavy metal toxicity or not, I recommend the following protocol to keep heavy metal accumulation to a minimum. Once you realize that heavy metals are in almost everything, you will also realize that you need to be proactive in detoxing and not accumulating more of it.

You will probably need to work with a health professional on this, as it can become tricky and quite uncomfortable. Even if you have never had a silver mercury filling placed in your teeth, you should still be evaluated to rule out the heavy metal factor contributing to your imbalance. Heavy metals are unknowingly passed to our children in utero (do any of your parents have mercury fillings or root canals?), from food (especially high mercury fish and foodstuff treated with pesticides, antibiotics and hormones), paints, and vaccines.

1. If you have any silver mercury fillings in your teeth, have them replaced. Make sure

to work with a qualified holistic dentist who knows the proper protection protocol when your silver mercury fillings are drilled out. Otherwise you may expose yourself to massive amounts of toxic mercury vapor causing a tremendous exposure and dire consequences. You can find information at this website: http://iaomt.org/. I would still ask questions of the particular practitioner that you are considering to make sure they are doing the right thing for your protection.

Also, reconsider the use of vaccines. Many have mercury (thimerosol) and aluminum added as a preservative.

2. Integrate chlorophyll rich drinks into your diet. Green juices are made from green superfoods- foods like barley grass, spirulina and other chlorophyll rich foods. These superfoods are packed with the vitamins and minerals that you need for detoxifying and rebuilding your immune system.

Chlorophyll from green foods supports intestinal and liver health, improves oxygen delivery by the blood, and assists elimination of certain toxins and heavy metals. It will inhibit absorption of environmental pollutants like dioxin and also help your body excrete many poisons and pollutants quicker. The high antioxidant level can slow aging by combating free radical damage. It has even been shown to repair DNA!

Chlorophyll not only enhances oxygen transport in your body, it is a top nutrient for balancing your body's pH by helping to reduce acidity. Also, maintaining a good body pH is so important in fighting off infections and inflammation. Low-grade acidosis may not only contribute to fatigue but other health concerns as well, including kidney stones and lower growth hormone levels, which lead to more body fat and loss of lean muscle mass.

Green juices are easily made from juicing organic vegetables or by adding any liquid to a dehydrated green juice powder. There are plenty of different brands of green juice powder at the health food store. So read the labels to find one that you feel is best for you with no allergenic additives. The powders are easy to work with as they mix easily into juice, smoothies or protein drinks. This makes it fairly palatable and simple to use. You have no excuse not to do this. Personally, I feel my daily green juice is more important than any multivitamin. If I miss a few days of green juice consumption, I not only feel worse, but I actually start craving them. When your body gets used to a higher energy level of health, it is hard to go backwards to where you were before. I can feel the vitality boost soon enough when green drinks are added back into my daily diet.

It is important to keep in mind that the health benefits of juicing are different than those received from eating green vegetables. Juice nutrients are much more easily absorbed, tolerated and utilized by the cells of your body than eating the whole vegetable with fiber. Both are healthful but juicing is a great deal more nutrient dense for the purposes of detoxing and rebuilding.

3. Ingest foods rich in phytoestrogens. They are found in flax seeds, sprouted beans, some fruits and vegetables. Phytoestrogens bind to the estrogen sites preventing the xenoestrogens from being bound. Do avoid soy products (tofu, soy milk, etc.) as there is much controversy on its side effects from over consumption.

4. Eat tons of cruciferous vegetables. (Preferably raw, fermented or lightly steamed). This would include cabbage, broccoli, brussel sprouts, and kale. They are rich in indole-3-carbinole. This converts to di-indolyl-methane (DIM). DIM then

induces certain enzymes in the liver to block the production of toxic estrogens and improves the production of the beneficial forms. If you have a hypothyroid condition, you should consult a qualified practitioner for guidance, since overconsumption of raw cruciferous foods may exacerbate an underactive thyroid.

5. Avoid caffeine as some studies show that it can boost estrogen levels. It is found in many foods: coffee, tea, chocolate, most sodas and even some analgesics. Please read labels carefully.

6. Avoid foods that have been treated with hormones or pesticides. These are both xenoestrogenic. Eat organic as much as possible.

7. Avoid the excessive use of lavender essential oil. It has been implicated as a xenoestrogen.

*   **Use natural personal care products.**

There are thousands of products on the market labeled as personal care products that could kill you if you use them too much. Hard to believe but poisoning incidents with cosmetics/products for personal care represent approximately 9% of all inquiries to the Poisons Control Center in the United States. (This is closely followed by 8.6% for household cleaners.) I would venture to say that these incidents are probably severe allergic reactions (anaphylaxis) or ingestion (child ingests lipstick or such).

Personal products mostly include shampoos, makeup, deodorants, baby powders and hair spray. The list is literally endless. Each of these usually has a petroleum base, heavy metal (aluminum, mercury) or a noxious chemical (sodium lauryl sulfate). Remember what the oil spills in our oceans did to our fish and birds? That's what petroleum products do to our skin. They make the surface of our skin nice and soft but it prevents the cells from actually breathing. It is like wrapping your skin in plastic wrap. Not a pretty picture. Plus petroleum products will draw out the fat soluble vitamins from your skin which will ultimately make you and your skin age faster.

Our rule of thumb is: if it is toxic to ingest, then don't put it on your lips, skin or elsewhere. This is the same story that we already discussed with fluoride.

If you are looking for natural substitutes for personal care products, a little research on the internet will provide many. An excellent resource is www.earthclinic.com.

- **Continuously detoxify and prevent further poison accumulation.**

The human brain forms and develops over a long period of time as compared to other organs, with rapid brain growth continuing throughout childhood. The blood brain barrier is not fully developed until much later in life, and even then, many toxins can still go through this barrier affecting the brain neurons. Heavy metals are definitely at the top of this list. In utero, the fetus has been found to get significant exposure to toxic substances through the maternal blood and across the placenta, with fetal metal toxicity levels often being higher than that of the mom. Also significant is that toxicity exposure has been found in children who were breastfed.

The incidence of neurotoxic or immune reactive conditions such as Multiple Sclerosis, Alzheimer's, ADD, ADHD, autism, learning disabilities, asthma, allergies etc., has been increasing, sometimes exponentially, in recent years. Being labeled with these dis-eases, given a medicine and being written off with a chronic lifelong diagnosis of "incurable", is not what anyone wants to hear.

As I have mentioned before, just because the conventional medical field has no solutions, this doesn't mean that they don't exist. It is up to us to be proactive for our own health. Educate ourselves and take steps to secure our own future. Waiting for someone else to heal us is basically giving away our power. Remember you were born a lot healthier than you are presently. So, what happened between then and now?

Basically, you became a holding tank for all the poisons that you were exposed to over your entire lifetime. Remember that these pollutants are everywhere, mostly insidiously hidden in the guise of food, medicine and a comfortable lifestyle.

So to break this cycle of accumulating any more, here is what you need to do. Daily, weekly and continuously, detoxify for the rest of your life. Just as you would brush your teeth as a daily habit, you need to detoxify daily.

1. Take soaking salt or clay baths once or twice a week. Baths are wonderfully healing, and it is easy to make your own homemade salt baths. Hot water relaxes the muscles and

dilates the blood vessels, allowing more oxygen throughout the body. As more oxygen moves through the cells, you will automatically remove toxic wastes from the cells. The salt in the bath draws toxins out of the body to the skin's surface through a simple process of osmosis.

Using one half to one full cup of salt (Epsom, sea or Himalayan) will allow for detoxification. Other salts—all highly alkaline and cleansing—used in baths, include baking soda and clay. All are good in different ways, so you should try to vary the salts in your baths. Notice how you feel after each, and do what makes you feel the best.

2. Try rebounding on a mini trampoline. When you use a rebounder, it promotes circulation through the body's lymphatic system. The toxins are moved to the lymph ducts, which transport the toxins to the kidney and liver, and ultimately out of the body. It is a great fun exercise and if done daily, will serve as an insurance policy against many serious diseases. Rebounding is a good way to get even the most sedentary person moving. It is not only great exercise, but it is fun too. Sometimes I will do it with my favorite music or even while watching TV (if you

must). The blood will flow, the toxins will go and the brain will glow! (Funny how I just came up with that).

3. Do oil pulling daily. Oil pulling is a simple Ayurvedic healing process for the oral cavity and the entire human body. It is great for acute infections of the mouth but therapeutic for chronic health challenges. One may have to practice oil pulling for months before long term results are noticed. It is valuable for purifying and strengthening the body. According to Ayurveda, organ meridians are present throughout the oral cavity. The tongue, in particular, has key meridian points similar to the hands, feet, ears and teeth.

Every organ in the human body is connected to other parts of the human body. We also know that each tooth and different parts of the tongue are associated with specific organs. When you heal teeth and its environmental structures, the meridian associated organs will also heal. Oil pulling will pull toxins from the mucus membranes of the mouth via the meridian system allowing for a complete body detoxification.

Traditionally, oil pulling has been used with sesame

or sunflower oils, but has been modified recently to accommodate other oils and their healing properties. For general health purposes, I am partial to coconut oil due to its antibacterial, antifungal and antiviral properties. The oral cavity is full of bacteria, fungi and viruses. Coconut oil pulling is great at keeping a healthy mouth and has also been shown to remineralize tooth enamel. (Now we really have no reason to keep fluoride in our system.)

It is also a cooling oil and will work wonders on pulling out heat /congestion and assist in relieving infections, fevers, burns, cold sores, oral herpes outbreaks, and reduce overgrowth of Candida in the mouth. It may also alleviate the pain associated with these oral conditions. This is how you use it:

How to Oil Pull:
After thoroughly cleaning your teeth and gums, place approximately one tablespoon of organic virgin coconut oil in your mouth. The oil is put in the mouth, with chin tilted up, and slowly swished, sucked, chomped and pulled through the teeth for 15–20 minutes.

The oil changes from oily consistency to thin, white milky foam before spitting it out. If the oil is still oily, it has not been pulled long enough.

Spit it into the garbage or toilet. Do not spit the oil down the sink, as the oil will eventually clog your drain. Thoroughly rinse and wash your mouth with normal tap water.

Oil pulling should be done at least once a day, preferably in the morning on an empty stomach. No more than twice. Time constraints may be a factor, so it is a good thing to do in the shower, while reading, doing housework, etc.

There are other benefits to coconut oil pulling:

- May stop tooth decay due to its antibacterial effects
- Will support periodontal health, may reverse gum infections
- Will help eradicate yeast infections in the mouth due to the presence of caprylic acid
- May whiten your teeth
- Can facilitate absorption of calcium by the body; it helps in getting strong teeth and bones

Sunflower, sesame, olive and flax oils have been used with varying results. Best to try each of these oils for a short time period to see which feels best for your specific condition.

4. Do dry body brushing. Dry skin brushing is one of the healthiest self-help methods available to us today. The best part is that it takes seconds to do, can be done in the comfort of your own home, and is painless and cost free.

Dry skin brushing promotes movement of the lymphatic system which can become stagnant or thick due to overload of toxins in the body or during an intense detoxification cleansing program. It will give your lymph system a kick start and help you feel refreshed and invigorated. Circulation improves, your skin becomes softer and healthier, and whole body wellness is enhanced. Your level of immunity increases and even common infections can be prevented.

How to Dry Skin Brush:

1. Purchase a natural, NOT a synthetic, bristle brush.

2. Purchase a brush with a long handle, so that you are able to reach all areas of your body.

3. Skin brushing should be performed once a day, preferably first thing in the morning. If you are feeling ill, please do it twice a day until you feel better.

4. Skin brushing should be performed prior to your bath or shower and your body should be dry. It might even be smart to do it while standing in the tub, so that dry skin can be washed away in the shower afterward.

5. Begin brushing your skin in long sweeping strokes starting from the bottom of your feet upwards, and from the hands towards the shoulders, and on the torso in an upward direction. Always brush towards the lymph glands so that toxins can be more easily released. Try and brush several times in each area, over-lapping as you go. *Note:* Major lymph glands are located under the jaw, at the underarms and in the groin areas. If this is too difficult to remember, then just brush towards the heart and 90% of the time you will be going in the right direction.

6. Avoid sensitive areas and anywhere the skin is broken. If anything hurts when you do it, then avoid those areas or do it gently until it becomes more tolerable.

For a thorough lymphatic cleansing, perform skin brushing daily for a minimum of three months.

Please do not skin brush if you have any varicose

veins, painful rashes or open wounds.

Skin is the largest organ in the human body. It is responsible for one fourth of the body's detoxification, most of it through sweat. It eliminates two pounds of waste acids each day. So for those of us who are trying to be our healthiest, it would make sense to daily incorporate this simple detoxification technique.

Although not as popular, we have found that wet body brushing can be effective as well. It can be done in the shower or while soaking in a warm salt bath.

* * *

Building on a vibration of love, self-nurturance and wholesome foods, should culminate in an outcome more powerful than just exercise and vitamin supplements alone. Removing toxins from my body and home was, by far, the most important thing I did to regain my health. I still exercised and ate right, but that just kept me "sort of okay." Feeling amazing with vibrant health is so much better.

Our environment is so critical to regaining and maintaining excellent health. Do not underestimate it. If you are in a bad situation physically or emotionally, you need to make a shift. Not only will you heal yourself, but you can be sure that you will be setting an example for someone else. I never knew the impact my own health story had on others until years later when clients would seek me out, specifically because I had survived the debilitating and deadly effects of Lyme disease.

As the Nike logo says: *Just do it!*

Now What?

Faith is taking the first step, even when you don't see the whole staircase.
        -Martin Luther King Jr.

Everything that I have discussed, includes my basic do- it-yourself list for regaining health. There is always more that can be done and I would advise everyone reading this to stay fully conscious and further explore the many other aspects of preventing and removing everyday emotional, mental and physical poisons from your environment, your mind and your body.

Be proactive. Take back your power and do one new health promoting activity daily. Habits happen through day by day continuous repetition. If you can shower regularly, you certainly can soak in a salt bath regularly.

Start today and build from there. By empowering yourself, and taking the first step, you will set into motion a bigger chain reaction of continuing daily improved health.

When we realize that conventional sheeple (people behaving as sheep) mentality got us into this mess of pitiable habits and health, then we will step into our own glory, be our own advocate, and reclaim our birthright of glorious health.

Shifting your health starts with you. Believe that you can be healed. Be proactive in making it so, and you will be. It worked for me and it can for you.

You, as much as anybody in the entire universe, deserve your love and affection.
                          - Siddhārtha Gautama

We are all one. By healing ourselves, we will heal others. Be the change you wish to see in the world; starting now.

Blessings of good health for all. Namaste.

Made in the USA
Middletown, DE
17 April 2023

28726943R00046